M000219325

Tips for Aging at Home

Tips for Aging at Home

Doing What Matters to You

Laura N. Gitlin, PH.D., FGSA, FAAN
Sarah L. Szanton, PH.D., ANP, FAAN
Jill Roth, RN, BSN
Allyson Evelyn-Gustave, OTR/L

CAMINO BOOKS, INC.
Philadelphia

Manufactured in the United States of America
1 2 3 4   22 21 20 19

Library of Congress Control Number: 2019012167

Cataloging-in-Publication data available from the Library of Congress, Washington, DC.

ISBN 978-1-68098-032-5
ISBN 978-1-68098-033-2 (ebooks)

Cover design: Jerilyn DiCarlo

This book is adapted from the original ABLE flipbook which was developed in a randomized trial (Advancing Better Living for Elders) supported by the National Institute on Aging (Grant #5RO1AG13687) and refined through other funding sources including The Eastern Pennsylvania-Delaware Geriatric Education Center (EPaD GEC; Grant #D31HP08834) and the Erickson Foundation. We acknowledge the initial role of Tracey Vause Earland, Ph.D., OTR/L, in identifying tips from ABLE studies.

This revised book has also been expanded to include the components of the CAPABLE program which has been funded by Robert Wood Johnson Foundation and the National Institute on Aging (Grant #R01AG040100).

This book is available at a special discount on bulk purchases for educational, business, and promotional purposes. For information write:

Publisher
Camino Books, Inc.
P.O. Box 59026
Philadelphia, PA 19102
www.caminobooks.com

Contents

Introduction

Carrying out everyday activities, such as getting dressed, bathing, or preparing meals, may be difficult for you. There are simple things to help you continue doing the activities you enjoy, like going to temple or church, visiting friends and family, or going shopping.

This book has tips on how to carry out daily activities you may value—safely and easily. Some tips may require small changes to your home. Most tips cost nothing. Some of the tools recommended, such as a jar opener, long-handled reacher, and pillbox, have a small cost. Some suggestions involve installing equipment in your house such as grab bars and railings, for which you may want to engage a handyperson.

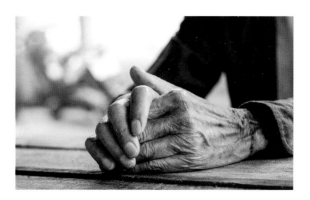

Most suggestions you can do on your own. Other tips need training from an occupational therapist or nurse.

Occupational therapists and nurses are uniquely trained to help people learn new strategies to make everyday tasks easier.

Who Are Occupational Therapists?

Occupational therapists look at a person's home and the way they live and carry out their day-to-day activities. They are experts at figuring out easier ways to do everyday tasks like cooking, cleaning, bathing, visiting friends and family, or shopping. Occupational therapists can help anyone, but they are especially helpful to people who have a hard time engaging in activities due to weakness or illness. An occupational therapist can work with you to identify your goals and how to achieve them safely.

Who Are Nurses?

Nurses promote health through preventing illness and injury, and decrease suffering by providing health care for individuals, families, and communities. A nurse can help you stay in your home by working with you to manage pain, mood, and medications, and to provide strength and balance and fall-prevention strategies.

Who Is a Handyperson?

A handyperson can be a man or a woman who is knowledgeable about home repairs and home modifica-

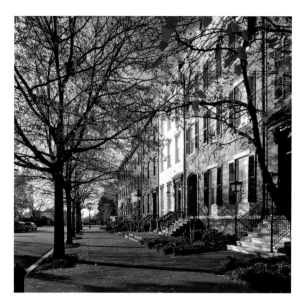

tions. Repairs that can help you do the things you want to might include patching holes in floors, installing new door locks, or fixing broken steps. Common home modifications may include installing grab bars in bathrooms and railings in stairwells. Other helpful and inexpensive improvements can include re-routing electrical cords, installing motion lights, and adding chain extensions to ceiling fans and lights.

How to Use This Tip Book

The tips in this book can help you:

- Do everyday activities safely.
- Do everyday tasks in small parts to make each part easier and less tiring.
- Decrease risk for falling.

Turn to the section that you are interested in. Read the suggestions on that page and see which ones work for you. Keep in mind that everyone is different and that all of the tips listed might not work for you. You may need to change a tip to fit your situation.

Some people find it helpful to write down the tips that they have tried and how they worked. There is a page for you to keep track of what works for you at the end of the book.

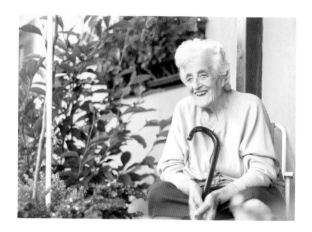

The suggestions in this book come from research with older adults, people with physical disabilities, and the best clinical practices of occupational therapists and nurses.

The tips offered in this book were tested as part of a randomized clinical trial, Project ABLE (Advancing Better Living for Elders), and expanded on in the CAPABLE program. Older adults who participated in these studies worked with occupational therapists, nurses, and physical therapists (in ABLE) and used the tips in this book. Participants reported fewer difficulties and more confidence with their daily activities and decreased fear of falling. Those who participated in the ABLE program lived longer than other older adults. Most of the CAPABLE participants were able to care for themselves more easily and were less depressed.

The authors intend this book for guidance, not to replace advice or directions given by your primary health care provider, occupational therapist, nurse, or other health professional. Some recommendations

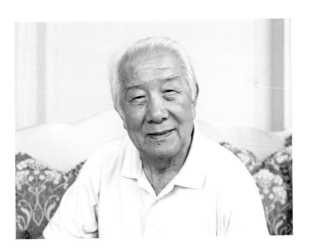

may require additional instruc-
tion from a therapist. Because this
book contains suggested tips, the
authors disclaim liability for any
injuries resulting in connection with
their use.

Dressing and Grooming

Tips for Getting Dressed and Groomed

☐ Keep everyday items in easy-to-reach places, such as clothes on coat hooks or on a lower rod in a closet.

☐ Wear sturdy shoes that have a firm grip but do not stick on the floor.

☐ Use a long-handled shoehorn, sock aid, dressing stick, or reacher to put on socks and shoes.

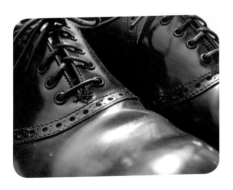

- ☐ Use long-handled combs and brushes for your hair, and extended toothbrushes to brush your teeth.
- ☐ Sit to do grooming tasks (washing face, shaving, brushing teeth) when you can.
- ☐ Wear clothes that fit. Avoid loose, flowing clothes that you could trip on.
- ☐ Wear clothing that is easy to put on and take off, such as elastic waistbands, sports bras, and Velcro™ instead of shoe laces.

Preparing Meals

Best Tips in the Kitchen

☐ Take time and move slowly while working in the kitchen.

☐ Keep cooking items close by.

☐ Hang items on peg boards, use a lazy Susan or coat hooks.

☐ Use lightweight pots, pans, and food containers.

☐ Use a baby stroller or cart to transport heavy items like cans, pots, and pans.

☐ Sit on a sturdy chair while cooking whenever you can.

☐ Sit instead of stand to reach for items on the floor or in a low cabinet.

☐ Plan to cook in small steps; for example, chop vegetables one day, and the next day have someone carry heavy cans or pans for you.

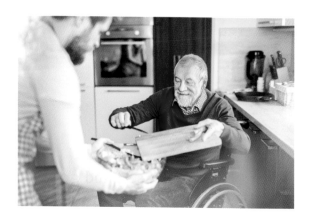

☐ Avoid standing on a chair to reach items that are high up. Instead, use a sturdy step stool with a hand rail.

☐ Hold on to a secure surface like a counter top for balance when reaching or standing.

☐ Keep one hand free when carrying items to brace yourself if you lose your balance.

☐ Keep your microwave in a place that is easy to reach.

Bathing and Using the Toilet

Best Tips in the Bathroom

☐ Use a raised toilet seat and grab bars to make using the toilet easier.

☐ Use a tub bench, shower chair, grab bars, and a hand-held shower hose to make bathing easier and safer.

☐ Use a long-handled sponge or soap on a rope to help you wash up.

☐ Install grab bars on the side of tub or shower walls.

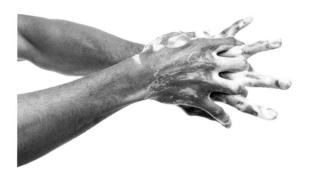

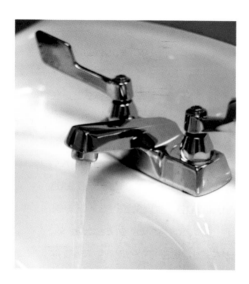

☐ Keep frequently used items in easy-to-reach places.

☐ Put a non-skid mat or bath safety strips in the bathtub. Have non-sliding rugs on the floor

☐ Light the hallway from bedroom to bathroom at night. Use night-lights, motion lights, or keep a light on all night.

☐ Set the hot water heater at less than 110 degrees Fahrenheit.

☐ Use lever-style sink handles instead of twist or pull handles.

☐ Have soap, washcloth, shampoo, and towel in the bathroom before beginning to bathe.

☐ Plan to sit after a bath in case you get light-headed.

☐ Stand on a level, non-slip surface when bending or reaching. Keep one hand on something sturdy like a counter top.

☐ Change glass shower or tub doors to a shower rod and curtain.

Changes for Specific Concerns

Tips and Tools for Poor Eyesight

☐ Use reading glasses or a magnifying glass with a light.

☐ Use talking appliances such as a clock, glucometer, alarms, timers, or sensors.

☐ Get large-print books and magazines or Talking Books from the Library for the Blind.

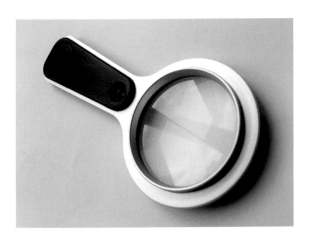

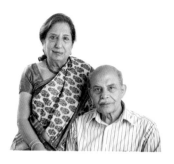

☐ Get labels with large print on your medicine bottles (ask your pharmacist).

Tools for Weak Hand s and Arms

☐ Electric can opener, jar opener, and bag cutter.

☐ Pill boxes and easy-to-open pill bottles (non-childproof).

☐ Pot and bowl holders.

☐ Cutting boards that hold food so you can cut with one hand.

☐ Items that attach to the hands to help you hold tools and utensils.

☐ Lever handles in place of door knobs.

☐ Button aids and zipper pulls.

☐ Key turners.

**Tips and Tools for Poor Balance
and Weak Legs**

☐ Raise furniture and appliances to waist height, including counter tops, washer, and dryer.

☐ Raise toilet seat or toilet frame.

☐ Add a cushion on a chair or use an electronic lift chair.

☐ Chair risers can raise chairs, beds, and sofas.

☐ Use a shower chair or tub bench.

☐ Install handles, railings, and banisters inside and outside.

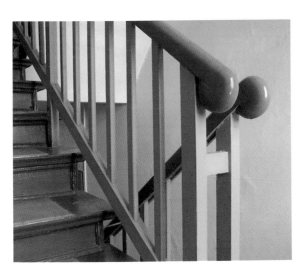

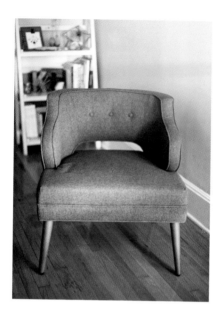

☐ Consider removing doors or widening doorways to 36 inches.

☐ Put a chair to rest on in every room.

Saving Energy

Take Time

- ☐ Avoid rushing. For example, do not rush to answer the door or telephone.
- ☐ Carry a cell phone or portable phone all of the time.
- ☐ Plan ahead before you begin a task. Gather everything needed for each step before starting the task.

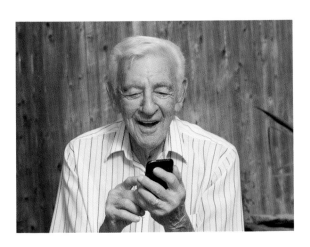

☐ Break down tasks into small steps. Decide if some steps can be done later or eliminated.

EXAMPLE: *When taking clothes from washer to dryer, do not shake out the clothes. Tumbling in the dryer will untangle the clothes.*

Arrange Your Home to Save Energy

☐ Raise chairs, sofas, and toilet seats by using extra padding, chair risers, and raised toilet seats. It is easier to get up from a high seat.

☐ Keep items in easy-to-reach places on peg boards, a lazy Susan, or coat hooks.

☐ Keep supplies you need for a task in a container. Carry supplies from one place to another, such as cleaning items, in a small basket with a handle.

☐ Organize items in a closet or cabinet with shelves and small containers.

☐ Have more than one cleaning tool on different levels: for example, have two vacuum cleaners, one for upstairs and one for downstairs. In this way you don't have to carry it up and down the steps.

EXAMPLE: Have extra cleaning supplies, such as window cleaners and scouring pads, to keep upstairs and downstairs to help you save steps and physical energy.

☐ Keep emergency numbers and important information handy. This saves steps when you suddenly need the information.

Planning Ahead Can Save Energy

☐ Make a detailed schedule for the day.

☐ Spread activities throughout the whole day.

☐ Take frequent rests.

☐ Rest before doing activities that make you tired, such as visiting grandchildren or going shopping.

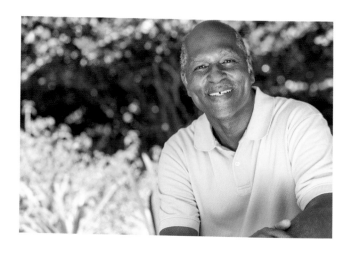

☐ Rest at times during the day when you usually get tired.
  EXAMPLE: *If you get tired in the late afternoon, plan to rest at that time.*

☐ Use cleaning supplies that make chores easier and safer. For example, use floor cleaners you do not have to rinse and tub sprays you do not have to scrub.

☐ Place items at waist height when working. This makes work such as cooking and folding laundry easier.

☐ Do as many jobs as possible in one place. While chopping vegetables

at the kitchen table, wipe off the
table and organize the mail.

☐ Avoid doing tasks that cannot be
broken down into sections, like
cooking complicated meals.

Moving Safely Around Your Home

Tips to Make Tasks Easier

☐ Use a baby stroller, cart, containers, bags, and buckets to carry things.

☐ Use lightweight items to cook and store food.

☐ Use the telephone and computer for errands if possible.

☐ Get groceries and medicines delivered to your home.

☐ Use small electric appliances, such as hand mixers, rather than stir by hand.

☐ Use a walker that has a basket, bag, or tray to keep items that you need close by.

Tips to Make Your Home Safer

☐ Remove tripping hazards.
  —Repair broken steps and loose carpeting.
  —Light stairways, steps, and hallways.
  —Watch your pets or tie them up while walking.
  —Keep floors, stairways, and hallways clear.
  —Avoid using area rugs, or secure them with non-slip rug pads.
☐ Light up your house.
  —Keep all rooms well lit. Shadows can make it hard to see things in your way.
  —When walking from a dark to a bright area, move slowly, take your time.
  —Light the path from bedroom to bathroom at night. Use night lights.
  —Use lamp shades to cut down the glare.

Tips for Walking

☐ Think about the way you walk.

☐ Stand upright while walking.

☐ Look forward to see in front of you.

☐ Outdoors, look for uneven sidewalks, curbs, and cracked sidewalks.

☐ When going up or down steps, take one step at a time and hold on to a railing.

☐ Walk more slowly during bad weather.

☐ Be aware of slippery wet surfaces.

Tips to Use Your Body Better

☐ Roll or slide heavy items instead of carrying.

☐ If you have to carry bags, such as grocery bags, hold them close to your body so you don't hurt your back. Do not over-pack your bags.

☐ Do not move your arms in a fast motion, such as sweeping with a broom. Keep all movements slow and steady.

☐ When using your hands, keep your elbows on a sturdy surface like a table or counter top.

☐ Sit to work whenever possible.

☐ When getting out of bed, roll to one side and use your arms to push your body up to a sitting position while dropping your legs to the floor.

☐ When getting out of a chair, scoot to the edge and use both hands to help push yourself up to a standing position.

Preventing Falls

Tips for Better Balance

☐ Sit, instead of stand, to reach for items on the floor or in a low cabinet.

☐ Keep one hand free when carrying items. If you lose your balance, your free hand can steady you.

☐ Face the direction you want to bend or reach to help you keep your balance.

☐ Stand on a level, non-slip surface while bending or reaching. Do not stand on a chair or throw rug.

☐ Exercise:

—Getting stronger will improve your balance.

—Tai Chi is one exercise that helps older adults have better balance. Look for a class near you.

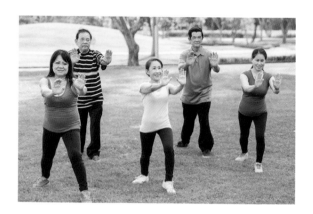

☐ Change positions slowly:
—When you get out of bed, sit on the side of the bed until you feel safe to stand.
—Before walking, take a moment to stand, holding on to something sturdy like a couch or counter top, until you feel safe to move.
☐ Drink water.
—Dehydration can make people dizzy.
—Ask your healthcare provider how much water you can drink every day.

Tips to Prevent Falls

- ☐ Get your vision and hearing checked.
    - —Get your eyesight checked every 1–2 years.
    - —Get your hearing checked every 3–4 years.
- ☐ Use a reacher, or a step stool with a handrail, when reaching items up high.
- ☐ Add banisters or railings on all stairs, inside and outside. Make all railings sturdy.

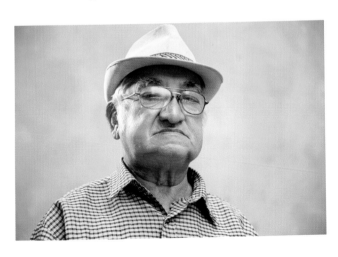

☐ Hold on to something sturdy for balance, such as a countertop, when reaching or standing.

☐ Wear clothes that fit and are easy to put on and take off, for example clothes with elastic waists or Velcro™ closures.

— Loose, flowing clothes could make you trip.

☐ Cut back on caffeine—coffee, tea, soda.

— Caffeinated drinks make you dehydrated, which can make you lightheaded.

— Caffeinated drinks can make you rush to the bathroom, which can cause falling.

☐ Keep your bones strong.

— Vitamin D makes your bones stronger. Ask your healthcare provider if you should take Vitamin D.

— Sit in the sun, without sunscreen, for 10 minutes every day.

- ☐ Control your urine so you do not rush and fall. (See the tips in the chapter "Controlling Urine.")
- ☐ Control blood sugar.
  - —High and low blood sugar can cause weakness, confusion, numbness in your feet, and frequent urination.
- ☐ Ask your healthcare provider or pharmacist to look at your medications to see if any of your medicines can cause you to fall.
- ☐ Check your shoes.
  - —Wear sturdy shoes that have a firm grip but do not stick on the floor.
  - —Make sure your shoes are not worn out. Worn shoe heels may lead to falls.
  - —Wear slippers that fit securely.
  - —Wear shoes that use laces or Velcro™ to secure to your feet.
  - —Do not wear high heels.

☐ Keep wheelchairs, canes, walkers, and scooters in good shape. The rubber tips on your walker and canes should not be worn and the screws should be tight.

If You Do Fall

☐ Stay calm, try to relax, think about how you are feeling. Are you hurt?
☐ Before moving, plan how to get up from the floor.
   —Get on your hands and knees, all fours, close to sturdy furniture.
   —Pull yourself up into a chair and rest before standing up.

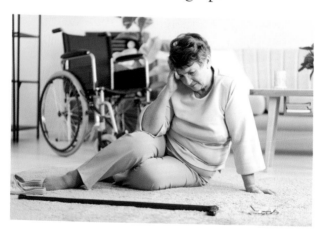

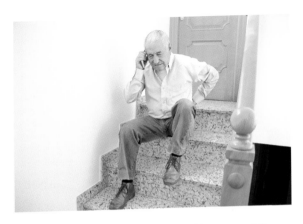

☐ Tell someone if you fall, even if
you think that you did not get
hurt.
—A family member or friend can
help you decide if you need to
go to the hospital.
—Your healthcare provider will
want to figure out what caused
your fall and will help you
decide if you need to go to the
emergency room or to the provider's office.

Improving Your Mood

☐ Pray or meditate.
— Many older adults find prayer or meditation gives comfort and hope.
☐ Participate in social activities.
— Go to church, mosque, temple, or your favorite gathering place.
— See your friends and family.
— Volunteer to help others.

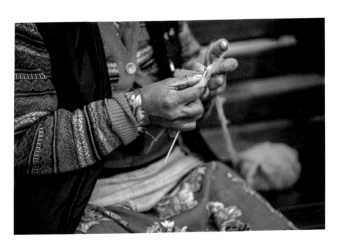

☐ Exercise and activity improve mood by decreasing pain and helping you get better sleep.
☐ Do simple exercises:
  —Walk (inside or outside).
  —Dance, standing or seated (even if it's by yourself).
  —Garden (start a window box or grow house plants).
  —Clean your house.
  —Swim or join a water aerobics class.
☐ Consider talk therapy.
  —Find a counselor through a community health clinic or your primary care provider.
☐ If you have diabetes, control your blood sugar.
  —High blood sugar can cause depression or "the blues."
☐ Control pain—chronic pain can make people depressed.
  —Control your pain before it gets bad.
  —Rest/relax.

   —Use ice/heat (see the chapter
      "Controlling Pain").
   —Take pain medication as
      prescribed.
   —Keep moving; sitting still makes
      you stiff.
☐ Eat a balanced diet of fruit, veg-
   etables, and whole grains.
☐ Get a good night's sleep.

Controlling Urine

Avoid Constipation

☐ When you are constipated, your intestines are full and press on the bladder.

—Drink more water. Not drinking enough can cause the stool to be hard, making it difficult to have a bowel movement.

—Eat more fiber found in fruit, vegetables, and high-fiber cereal. Fiber keeps stool soft.

—Exercise, move more.

Toileting

☐ Take time toileting.

—Sit, longer than usual, on the toilet to urinate until more urine comes out.

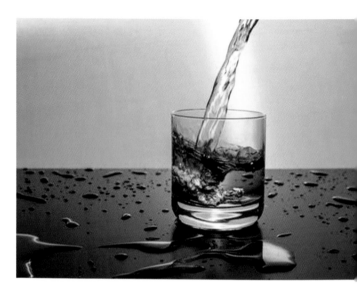

☐ Timed toileting
—Go to the bathroom every 2 hours whether you feel like you have to or not. In this way, you control your urine, it doesn't control you.

☐ Double toileting or "Sit, Stand, Sit":
—When you have to urinate, sit on the toilet.
—Then stand up for a few seconds and sit down again and urinate again.

Other Tips

☐ Cut back on caffeine.
— Drinks with caffeine include: coffee, tea, green tea, iced tea, and most dark sodas (such as Coke, Diet Coke, Pepsi, Diet Pepsi, and Mountain Dew).
— Caffeine makes you urinate or go to the bathroom more. Caffeine is a diuretic and irritates the bladder.
— Do not drink coffee, tea, and soda late in the afternoon or evening. When you avoid caffeine late in the day, you will have to go to the bathroom (urinate) less at night.

☐ If you have diabetes
— Control your blood sugar.
— High blood sugar can make you go to the bathroom more.

☐ Bladder infections:
— Bladder infections can feel like burning during urination and

make you go to the bathroom a lot.

—Always wipe from front to back after using the bathroom.

☐ Pelvic (vagina or penis) muscle exercises:

—Strengthen your pelvic or vaginal and penile muscles to have more control of your urine.

—To identify your pelvic muscles: While going to the bathroom, squeeze your vaginal or penile muscle and cut off your stream of urine. That is the muscle you are going to exercise.

—Do not do the exercises on the toilet.

—Do pelvic muscle exercises while watching TV.

—Squeeze your pelvic muscles and hold for 3 seconds, then release. Do this 10 times every day.

Controlling Pain

☐ Contact your provider if the pain continues or gets worse.

☐ Stop pain before it gets bad.

—Once people are in a lot of pain it is harder to stop.

—Start relieving pain when it is mild.

☐ Try using heat or cold.

—HEAT: Use a heating pad or a warm wet towel on the painful area.

—A heating pad can burn your skin if left on longer than 20 minutes.

—COLD: Use an ice pack or a bag of frozen vegetables on the painful area.

—Ice can burn your skin if left on longer than 20 minutes.

☐ Exercise and stay active; joints get
stiff when not in use.
  —Exercise your joints.
  —Walk (inside or outside).
  —Dance at home.
  —Garden.
  —Cook, clean, or do your laundry.
  —Swim or join a water aerobics
    class.
  —Try Tai Chi or a stretching class.

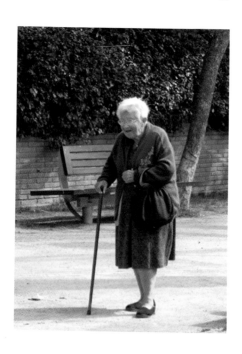

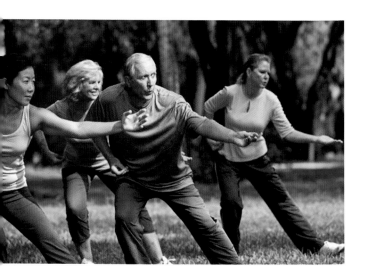

☐ Stop smoking.
  —Smoking can make arthritis
    worse.
☐ Listen to music.
☐ Pray or meditate.

Taking Medicine

Medication List

☐ Bring your medication list to your medical appointments and make changes as needed.

☐ Include herbal supplements, vitamins and over-the-counter medications on your medication list.

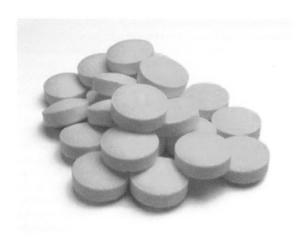

Right Medicine at the Right Time

☐ Check the name, time, and dose of medicine with your medication list before you take your medications.

☐ Tell your healthcare provider about any side effects you may be having.

☐ If you cannot see the information on your pill bottles:

—Ask your pharmacy to use large print on your medicine bottles.

—Use a magnifying glass to read the labels on your pill bottles.

☐ Ask your pharmacy to use easy-open tops on your pill bottles.

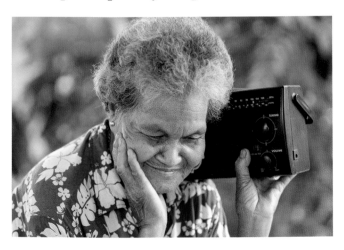

Remember to Take Medicines

☐ Try using a pillbox.

☐ Have a family member call to remind you to take your medicine.

☐ Try a medication reminder alarm to remind you to take your medicines.

Over-the-Counter Medicines

☐ Many over-the-counter medicines contain several different medications.

☐ Read the medication labels carefully, especially the ingredients.

☐ Ask the pharmacist what other medicines are in the medicines that you are buying.

☐ Tell your primary care provider about all new medications and vitamins that you start.

Hard-to-Swallow Pills

☐ Take pills with thicker liquid or food, such as milk, applesauce, or yogurt.

☐ Ask a pharmacist if you can crush or cut your pills.

☐ Ask if your medicine comes in a smaller-size pill or liquid.

Running Out of Medicines

☐ Get your pills refilled before you run out.

☐ Many medicines have serious side effects if stopped suddenly.

☐ Talk to your healthcare provider before stopping any medications.

Where to Get More Information

Be sure to record local contact information in the chart below.

Condition	Organization	Contact	Local #
All conditions	National Institute on Aging, Age Pages	www.nih.gov/nia/health 1-800-222-2225	
Arthritis	Arthritis Foundation	www.arthritis.org 1-800-283-7800	
Stroke	American Stroke Association	www.stroke.org 1-800-787-6537	
Diabetes	American Diabetes Association	www.diabetes.org 1-800-DIABETES	
Parkinson's Disease	National Parkinson's Foundation	www.parkinson.org 1-800-327-4545	
Lung diseases	American Lung Association	www.lungusa.org 1-800-LUNGUSA	
Osteoporosis	NIH Site on Osteoporosis and Related Bone Diseases	www.osteo.org 1-800-624-BONE	
Macular degeneration	Macular Degeneration Foundation	www.eyesight.org 1-888-633-3937	

Record of Tips Used

Use this form to record tips you have tried
and whether you found them helpful.

Tip	Date Tried	Helpful/ Not Helpful	Why?

Tip	Date Tried	Helpful/ Not Helpful	Why?

Also of interest to readers of
Tips for Aging at Home

A Caregiver's Guide to Dementia

Laura N. Gitlin, Ph.D.
Catherine Verrier Piersol, Ph.D., OTR/L

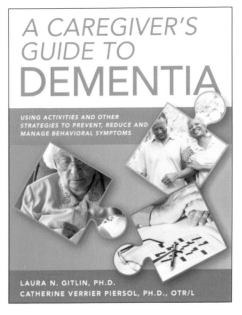

"The book consists of brief, straight-forward advice on managing a loved one whose brain has stopped keeping up with the demands of daily life."

—*The Washington Post*